BREAD MACHINE COOKBOOK

A Cookbook That Will Teach You How to Make The Best Use of The Bread Machine

Katlyn Williams

bread machine cookbook

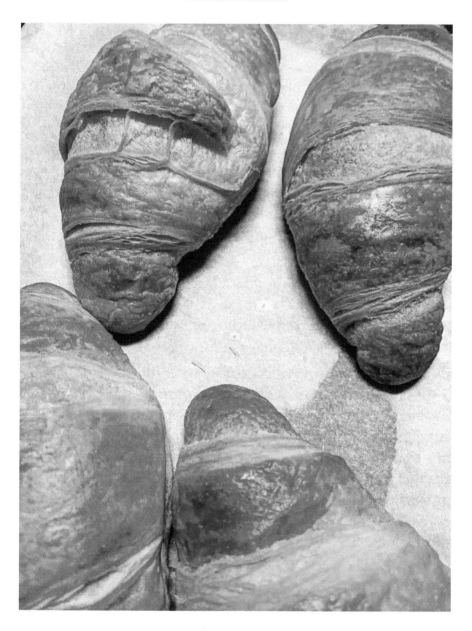

Table Of Contents

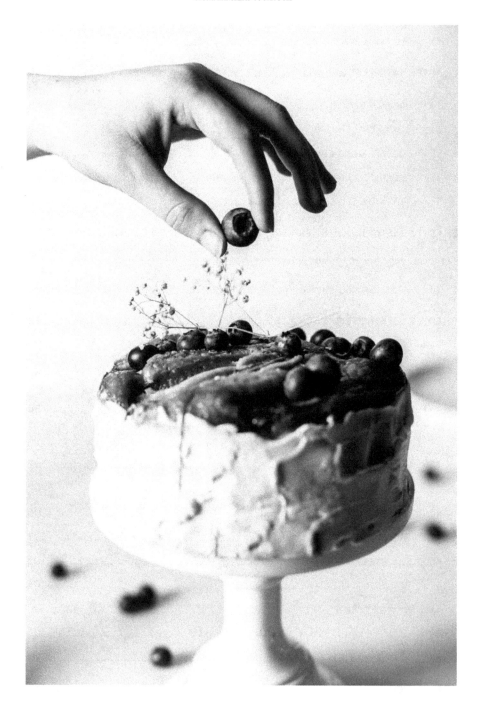

Introduction

Bread making machine, otherwise known as a bread maker, is a home-based appliance that transforms uncooked ingredients into bread. It is made up of a saucepan for bread (or "tin"), with one or more built-in paddles at the bottom, present in the center of a small special-purpose oven. This little oven is usually operated via a control panel via a simple in-built computer utilizing the input settings. Some bread machines have diverse cycles for various forms of dough — together with white bread, whole grain, European-style (occasionally called "French"), and dough-only (for pizza dough and formed loaves baked in a traditional oven). Many also have a timer to enable the bread machine to work without the operator's attendance, and some high-end models allow the user to program a customized period. To bake bread, ingredients are measured in a specified order into the bread pan (usually first liquids, with solid ingredients layered on top), and then the pan is put in the bread maker. The order of ingredients is important because contact with water triggers the instant yeast used in bread makers, so the yeast and water have to be kept separate until the program starts. It takes the machine several hours to make a bread loaf. The products are rested first and brought to an optimal temperature. Stir with a paddle, and the ingredients are then shaped into a loaf. Use optimal temperature regulation, and the dough is then confirmed and then cooked. When the bread has been baked, the bread maker removes the pan. Then leaving a slight indentation from the rod to which the paddle is connected. The finished loaf's shape is often regarded as unique. Many initial bread machines manufacture a vertically slanted towards, square, or cylindrical loaf that is significantly dissimilar from commercial bread; however, more recent units typically have a more conventional horizontal pan. Some bread machines use two paddles to form two lb. loaf in regular rectangle shape. Bread machine recipes are often much smaller than regular bread recipes. Sometimes standardized based on the machine's pan capacity, most popular in the US market is 1.5 lb. /700 g units. Most recipes are written for that capacity; however, two lb. /900 g units are not uncommon. There are prepared bread mixes, specially made for bread makers, containing pre-measured ingredients and flour and yeast, flavorings, and sometimes dough conditioners. Bread makers are also fitted with a timer for testing when bread-making starts. For example, this allows them to be loaded at night but only begin baking in the morning to produce a freshly baked bread for breakfast.

CHAPTER 1:

How to Use a Bread Machine?

Meet Your New Bread Machine

Hot golden crescents, freshly baked breakfast cakes, aromatic tea cakes, and delicious cakes to accompany your morning coffee. All of these can be cooked with a bread machine in minutes and with a little effort on your part. Also, these delicious and healthy baked goods can be made with the simplest and most common ingredients.

The only special thing you need to add is your love and creativity! As for the boring and routine tasks, such as baking, mixing, stirring, the bread machine will take care of them, leaving you the best and most enjoyable, that is, the choice of the recipe and the choice of ingredients. Isn't this a great way to enjoy the unique aroma and flavor of exactly the type of baked goods you need? Even if you're not good at using modern appliances, put your worries behind you because bread machines have simple, easy-to-use controls. They are fun and easy to use! Besides making fresh bread, they can also make and knead any type of dough, bake dough out of the box, and even make dough jam.

Main Ingredients

The ingredients needed for bread making are very simple: flour, yeast, salt, and liquid. There are other ingredients that add flavor, texture, and nutrition to your bread, such as sugar, fats, and eggs. The basic ingredients include:

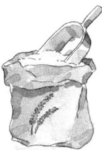

Flour is the foundation of bread. The protein and gluten in flour form a network that traps the carbon dioxide and alcohol produced by the yeast. Flour also provides simple sugar to feed the yeast, and it provides flavor, depending on the type of flour used in the recipe.

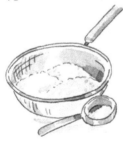

Yeast is a living organism that increases when the right amount of moisture, food, and heat are applied. Rapidly multiplying yeast gives off carbon dioxide and ethyl alcohol. When yeast is allowed to go through its life cycle completely, the finished bread is more flavorful. The best yeast for bread machines is bread machine yeast or active dry yeast, depending on your bread machine model.

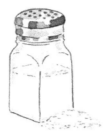

Salt strengthens gluten and slows the rise of the bread by retarding the action of the yeast. A slower rise allows the flavors of the bread to develop better, and it will be less likely the bread will rise too much.

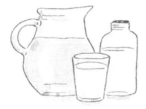

Liquid activates the yeast and dissolves the other ingredients. The most commonly used liquid is water, but ingredients such as milk can also be substituted. Bread made with water will have a crisper crust, but milk produces rich, tender bread that offers more nutrition and browns easier.

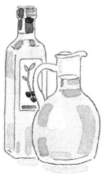

Oils and fats add flavor, create a tender texture, and help brown the crust. Bread made with fat stays fresh longer because moisture loss in the bread is slowed. This component can also inhibit gluten formation, so the bread does not rise as high.

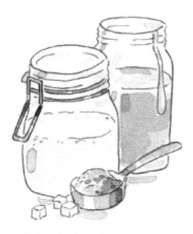

Sugar is the source of food for the yeast. It also adds sweetness, tenderness, and color to the crust. Too much sugar can inhibit gluten growth or cause the dough to rise too much and collapse. Other sweeteners can replace sugar, such as honey, molasses, maple syrup, brown sugar, and corn syrup.

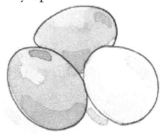

Eggs add protein, flavor, color, and a tender crust. Eggs contain an emulsifier, lecithin, which helps create a consistent texture, and a leavening agent, which helps the bread rise well.

CHAPTER 2:

Bread Machine Cycles

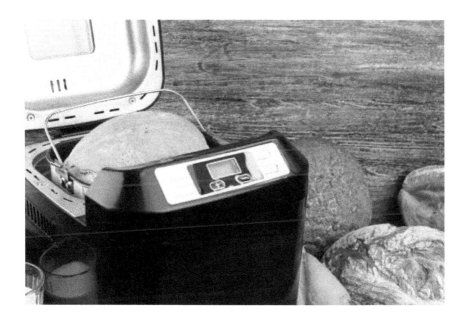

B read machines are a fantastic kitchen accessory to own. These small compact wonders have many options and settings for baking an assortment of bread masterfully. Once you become familiar with your bread machine's settings, the chance to create and experiment is endless. It is essential to know what each setting on your machine can deliver, making it easier to understand what function to use when it is time to bake your loaf. Being on a first-name basis with your bread machine will allow you to create flavorsome bread, making you wish that you had purchased the machine sooner! Bread machines can come in two different varieties.

Some brands hold specific settings that you cannot alter, so it is wise to follow the instruction manual when making different styles of bread to see which setting will be ideal. Whereas some bread machines come with basic settings with times and programming that you can alter. For instance, if you notice that the bread did not rise as you hoped for, you can extend the rising time. Now, let me help you understand the various cycles and settings that you can find on your bread machine.

Basic Cycle This setting is the most commonly used function of the bread machine, allowing you to create standard bread. This function generally runs for three to four hours, depending on the loaf size and style of bread. You can also use this setting when making bread using whole wheat flour.

Sweet Bread Cycle

This cycle, as the name suggests, is for bread that has higher sugar or fat content than standard bread. The setting is also used when ingredients such as cheese and eggs are used. This function allows the bread to bake at a lower temperature than other functions as the ingredients included may cause the crust to burn or darken in color.

Nut or Raisin Cycle

Though you can add ingredients such as nuts and dried fruit pieces into your pan, some machines tend to churn them too finely. The nut or raisin cycle is there to ensure that these ingredients stay relatively chunky, adding texture and sweetness to the bread. This function is ideal as it alerts the baker when it's time to add in the nuts or fruit pieces.

Whole Wheat Cycle

Whole wheat bread needs to be kneaded and churned longer than your standard loaves. That is why this cycle is perfect for bread that calls for this type of flour to be used. This function allows the bread to rise high enough and stops it from becoming too dense.

French bread Cycle

The majority of the bread from the Mediterranean regions such as Italy or France come out far better when using this function rather than the basic cycle. Many French styled loaves of bread hold none to very little sugar. Bread from these regions needs a longer rising time and a lower and longer temperature. This is so that it can create the textures and crusts we have grown to love and savor.

Dough Cycle

This is for those who make use of quick rise yeast in their bread recipes. The rapid cycle can take anywhere between 30 minutes to two hours of the basic bread cycle, saving you plenty of time. Note that the rapid bake cycle does vary from machine to machine.

Cake or Quick Cycle

This cycle ideal for recipes that contain no yeast, such as cakes. This a primary cycle to consider when making the store-bought cake and bread mixes. The bread machine does not knead the ingredients together like the other cycles. It only mixes the ingredients and bakes them. This cycle and baking time can also vary from one machine to the other.

Jam Cycle

Though bread is delicious served fresh from the bread machine, there is nothing quite as enjoyable as a warm slice of bread served with warm strawberry jam, one of my simple pleasures in life!

A jam cycle on a bread machine is an absolute treat. Quick tip, remember to finely dice your fruit before adding it into the bread machine for the best results. You can have a fresh pot of jam ready within one hour.

Time-Bake or Delayed Cycle

This is a novel setting that some bread machines have. It allows you to add the ingredients into the bread machine, then programs it to start baking at a time suited to you. This is a smart and useful function – thanks to it, there have been many days when the house has been awoken to the smell of fresh bread baking.

Word to the wise, bread that has milk or eggs as part of their ingredients should only be delayed for one to two hours to reduce issues with food-borne bacteria.

Crust Functionality

CHAPTER 3:

Bread Machine Techniques

The processes that occur in a bread machine are not that different than those you use when making bread by hand. They are just less work and mess. The primary techniques used in making bread from a bread machine are:

Mixing and resting.

The ingredients are mixed together well and then allowed to rest before kneading.

Kneading.

This technique creates long strands of gluten. Kneading squishes, stretches, turns, and presses the dough for 20 to 30 minutes, depending on the machine and setting.

First rise.

This is also called bulk fermentation. Yeast converts the sugar into alcohol, which provides flavor, and carbon dioxide, which provides structure as it inflates the gluten framework.

Stir down (1 and 2).

The paddles rotate to bring the loaf down and redistribute the dough before the second and third rise.

Second and third rise.

The second rise is about 15 minutes. At the end of the third rise, the loaf will almost double in size.

Baking.

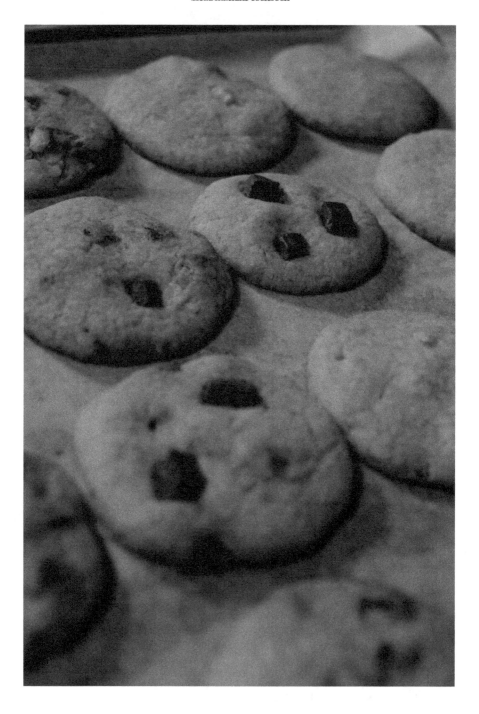

CHAPTER 4:

Famous Bread Recipes

## 1.	Texas Cheesy Bread

Preparation Time: 5 Minutes **Cooking Time:** 3 Hours

Servings: 12

Ingredients:

- 1 C. warm water
- 1 tsp. salt
- 2 tbsp. white sugar
- 1/2 C. shredded Monterey Jack cheese
- 6 tbsp. fresh chopped jalapeño peppers
- 3 C. bread flour
- 1/2 tbsp. active dry yeast

Directions:

1. In the bread machine pan, put all the ingredients in order as suggested by the manual.
2. Select the Regular Basic Bread cycle and press the Start button.

Nutrition:

Calories 152 kcal Fat 2 g Carbohydrates 27.3g Protein 5.5 g

Cholesterol 4 mg Sodium 220 mg

2.   Cinnamon Pinwheels

Preparation 1 Hour and 15 Minutes **Time:** 30 Minutes **Servings:** 24

Ingredients:

- 1 C. milk
- Two eggs
- 1/4 C. butter
- 4 C. bread flour
- 1/4 C. white sugar
- 1 tsp. salt
- 1 1/2 tsp. active dry yeast
- 1/2 C. chopped walnuts
- 1/2 C. packed brown sugar
- 2 tsp. ground cinnamon
- 2 tbsp. softened butter, divided
- 2 tsp. sifted confectioners' sugar, divided

Directions:

1. Add the milk, eggs, 1/4 C. of the butter, bread flour, sugar, salt, and yeast in order as suggested by the manual into the bread machine.

2. Select the Dough cycle and press the Start button.

3. After the completion of the cycle, place the dough onto a floured surface.

4. With your hands, thump down the dough and keep aside for about 10 minutes.

5. In a small bowl, add the brown sugar, walnuts, and cinnamon.

6. Place the dough onto a lightly floured surface and cut into two portions.

7. Now, roll each dough portion into a 9x14-inch rectangle.

8. Place 1 tbsp. of the softened butter over each dough rectangle evenly, followed by half of the walnut mixture.

9. Roll each dough rectangle, and with your fingers, pinch seams to seal the filling.

10. Place each loaf into a 9x5-inch greased loaf pan, seam side down

11. With plastic wraps, cover the pans and keep aside in a warm place for about 30 minutes.

12. Meanwhile, set your oven to 350 degrees F.

13. Place the bread in the oven for about 30 minutes. (In the last 10 minutes of the cooking, cover each loaf pan with foil pieces slightly to avoid over-browning).

14. Remove from the oven and keep onto a wire rack to cool for about 10 minutes.

15. Remove the bread loaves from pans and place them onto wire racks to cool completely before slicing.

16. Sprinkle top of each bread loaf with 1 tbsp. of the confectioners' sugar and cut into desired sized slices.

Nutrition: Calories 162 kcal Fat 5.5 g Carbohydrates 24.4g Protein 4.1 g Cholesterol 24 mg Sodium 129 mg

3. Garden Shed Bread

Preparation Time: 5 Minutes

Cooking Time: 25 Minutes

Servings: 12

Ingredients:

- 2/3 C. warm water
- 2/3 C. cottage cheese
- 2 tbsp. margarine
- 3 C. bread flour
- 1 tbsp. white sugar
- 1 tbsp. dry milk powder
- 1 tbsp. dried minced onion
- 1 tbsp. dill seed
- 1 tsp. salt
- 1 1/2 tbsp. active dry yeast

Directions:

1. In a bread machine pan, place all the ingredients in order as suggested by the manual.
2. Select the Basic Bread cycle and press the Start button.

Nutrition:

Calories 166 kcal Fat 3.1 g Carbohydrates   27.7g

Protein 6.6 g Cholesterol 2 mg

Sodium 270 mg

4. Bahamas Oat Bread

Preparation Time: 5 Minutes

Cooking Time: 25 Minutes

Servings: 10

Ingredients:

- 3/4 C. hot water
- 1/2 C. rolled oats
- 1 1/2 tsp. molasses
- 1 tbsp. butter
- 1/2 tsp. salt
- 1 1/2 C. bread flour
- 1 tbsp. active dry yeast

Directions:

1. In a container, add the hot water and oats and keep aside for about 2 minutes.
2. Add the molasses and butter and stir until well combined.
3. In a bread machine pan, add the oats mixture and remaining ingredients as suggested by the manual.
4. Select the White Bread cycle with the Light Crust and press the Start button.

Nutrition:

Calories 106 kcal Fat 1.8 g Carbohydrates   18.9g

Protein 3.5 g Cholesterol 3 mg

Sodium 126 mg

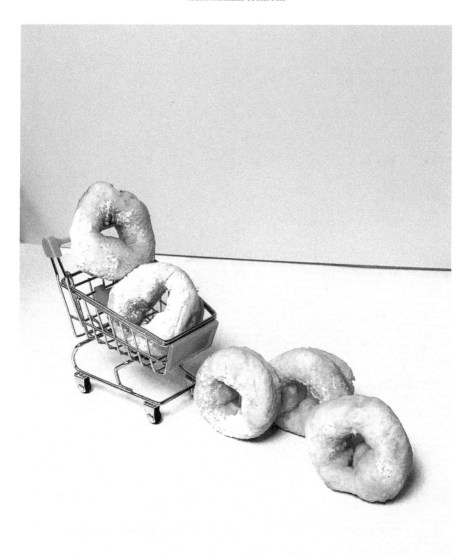

CHAPTER 5:

Italian Styled

5.   Sweet Easter Bread

Preparation Time: 5 minutes

Cooking Time: 35 minutes

Servings: 20 slices

Ingredients:

- teaspoons baking powder
- 1 cup water
- 1/2 cups almond flour
- 1/4 cup almond milk/ heavy cream
- cups whey isolate
- 1/2 cup sugar substitute
- 1/2 teaspoon salt
- 1/2 cup butter, melted
- teaspoons xanthan gum

Directions:

1   Add all ingredients to the Bread Machine.

2   Select Dough setting and press Start. Mix the ingredients for about 4-5 minutes. After that press stop button.

3   Smooth out the top of the loaf. Choose Bake mode and press Start. Let it bake for about 30 minutes.

4   Remove bread from the bread machine and let it rest for 10 minutes. Enjoy!

Nutrition:

150 calories

11.6 g fat

3.4 g total carb

9.6 g protein

6.   Zucchini Apple Fritter Bread

Preparation Time: 5 minutes

Cooking Time: 1 hour 10 minutes

Servings: 12 slices

Ingredients:

- teaspoons apple extract
- 1 medium zucchini peeled, seeded and chopped
- 1/4 cup Sorkin Gold
- 1/2 cup unsweetened almond milk
- 1 teaspoon cinnamon
- 1/2 teaspoon xanthan gum (optional)
- 1/2 cup low carb sugar substitute
- teaspoons baking powder
- 1/2 cup butter, softened
- 1/2 cup coconut flour
- eggs
- 1 cup almond flour
- Glaze:
- 2-3 tablespoons heavy cream
- 1/4 cup Sukrin Melis

Directions:

1   Add all ingredients to the Bread Machine.

2   Select Dough setting and press Start. Mix the ingredients for about 4-5 minutes. After that press stop button.

3   Smooth out the top of the loaf. Choose Bake mode and press Start. Let it bake for about 50 minutes.

4   For glaze, mix together 2-3 tablespoons heavy cream and 1/4 cup

5   Remove bread from the bread machine, let it rest a little and drizzle glaze over zucchini apple fritter bread.

Nutrition:

171 calories

15 g fat

6 g total carbs

4 g protein

7. Peanut Flour Bread

Preparation Time: 5 minutes

Cooking Time: 1 hour

Servings: 12

Ingredients:

- eggs
- 1 teaspoon baking powder
- 1/2 cup butter
- tsp guar gum/xanthan gum (optional)
- oz. cream cheese
- 1 1/3 cups peanut flour
- 3/4 cup low carb sugar substitute
- 1 teaspoon vanilla extract

Directions:

1 Add all ingredients to the Bread Machine.

2 Select Dough setting and press Start. Mix the ingredients for about 4-5 minutes. After that press stop button.

3 Smooth out the top of the loaf. Choose Bake mode and press Start. Let it bake for about 55 minutes.

4 Remove bread from the bread machine and let it rest for 10 minutes. Enjoy!

Nutrition: 152 calories 13 g fat 3 g total carbs

6g protein

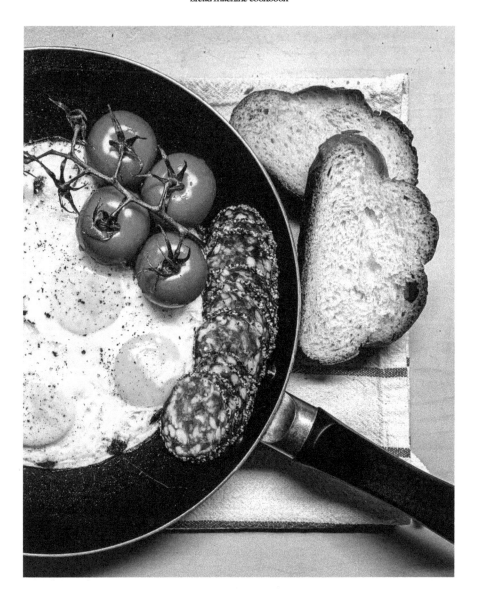

CHAPTER 6:

Special Bread Recipes

8. Grain-Free Chia Bread

Preparation Time: 5 Minutes

Cooking Time: 3 Hours

Servings: 12

Ingredients:

- 1 cup of warm water

- Three large organic eggs, room temperature

- 1/4 cup olive oil

- One tablespoon apple cider vinegar

- 1 cup gluten-free chia seeds, ground to flour

- 1 cup almond meal flour

- 1/2 cup potato starch

- 1/4 cup coconut flour

- 3/4 cup millet flour

- One tablespoon xanthan gum

- 1 1/2 teaspoons salt

- Two tablespoons sugar

- Three tablespoons nonfat dry milk

- Six teaspoons instant yeast

Directions:

1. Whisk wet ingredients together and place it in the bread maker pan.

2. Whisk dry ingredients, except yeast, together, and add on top of wet ingredients.

3. Make a well in the dry ingredients and add yeast.

4. Select the Whole Wheat cycle, light crust color, and press Start.

5. Allow cooling completely before serving.

Nutrition:

Calories: 375

Sodium: 462 mg

Dietary Fiber: 22.3 g

Fat: 18.3 g

Carbs: 42 g

Protein: 12.2 g

9.   Gluten-Free Brown Bread

Preparation Time: 5 Minutes

Cooking Time: 3 Hours

Servings: 12

Ingredients:

- Two large eggs, lightly beaten
- 1 3/4 cups warm water
- Three tablespoons canola oil
- 1 cup brown rice flour
- 3/4 cup oat flour
- 1/4 cup tapioca starch
- 1 1/4 cups potato starch
- 1 1/2 teaspoons salt
- Two tablespoons brown sugar
- Two tablespoons gluten-free flaxseed meal
- 1/2 cup nonfat dry milk powder
- 2 1/2 teaspoons xanthan gum
- Three tablespoons psyllium, whole husks
- 2 1/2 teaspoons gluten-free yeast for bread machines

Directions:

1. Add the eggs, water, and canola oil to the bread maker pan and stir until combined.

2. Whisk all of the dry ingredients except the yeast together in a large mixing bowl.

3. Add the dry ingredients on topmost of the wet ingredients.

4. Create a well in the center of the dry ingredients and add the yeast.

5. Set Gluten-Free cycle, medium crust color, and then press Start.

6. When the bread is done, lay the pan on its side to cool before slicing to serve.

Nutrition:

Calories: 201

Sodium: 390 mg

Dietary Fiber: 10.6 g

Fat: 5.7 g

Carbs: 35.5 g

Protein: 5.1 g

10.　Easy Gluten-Free, Dairy-Free Bread

Preparation Time: 15 Minutes

Cooking Time: 2 Hours and 10 Minutes

Servings: 12

Ingredients:

- 1 1/2 cups warm water
- Two teaspoons active dry yeast
- Two teaspoons sugar
- Two eggs, room temperature
- One egg white, room temperature
- 1 1/2 tablespoons apple cider vinegar
- 4 1/2 tablespoons olive oil
- 3 1/3 cups multi-purpose gluten-free flour

Directions:

1. Start with adding the yeast and sugar to the water, then stir to mix in a large mixing bowl; set aside until foamy, about 8 to 10 minutes.

2. Whisk the two eggs and one egg white together in a separate mixing bowl and add to the bread maker's baking pan.

3. Pour apple cider vinegar and oil into baking pan.

4. Add foamy yeast/water mixture to baking pan.

5. Add the multi-purpose gluten-free flour on top.

6. Set for Gluten-Free bread setting and Start.

7. Remove and invert the pan onto a cooling rack to remove the bread from the baking pan. Allow cooling completely before slicing to serve.

Nutrition:

Calories: 241

Sodium: 164 mg

Dietary Fiber: 5.6 g

Fat: 6.8 g

Carbs: 41 g

Protein: 4.5

CHAPTER 7:

Spice and Herb Bread

11. Awesome Rosemary Bread

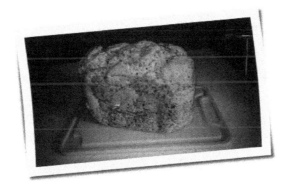

Preparation Time: 5 minutes

Cooking Time: 2 hours

Servings: 8 slices

Ingredients:

- 3/4 cup + 1 tablespoon water at 80 degrees F

- 1 2/3 tablespoons melted butter, cooled

- 2 teaspoons sugar

- 1 teaspoon salt

- 1 tablespoon fresh rosemary, chopped

- 2 cups white bread flour
- 1 1/3 teaspoons instant yeast

Directions:

1. Combine all of the ingredients to your bread machine, carefully following the instructions of the manufacturer.
2. Set the program of your bread machine to Basic/White Bread and set crust type to Medium.
3. Press START.
4. Wait until the cycle completes.
5. Once the loaf is ready, take the bucket out and allow the loaf to chill for 5 minutes.
6. Gently jiggle the bucket to take out the loaf.

Nutrition:

Total Carbs: 25g

Fiber: 1g

Protein: 4g Fat: 3g

Calories: 142

12. Original Italian Herb Bread

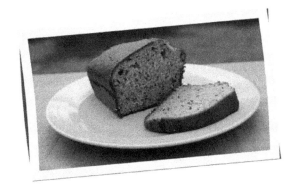

Preparation Time: 15 minutes

Cooking Time: 3 hours

Servings: 20 slices

Ingredients:

- 1 cup water at 80 degrees F
- ½ cup olive brine
- 1½ tablespoons butter
- 3 tablespoons sugar
- 2 teaspoons salt
- 5 1/3 cups flour
- 2 teaspoons bread machine yeast
- 20 olives, black/green
- 1½ teaspoons Italian herbs

Directions:

1. Cut olives into slices.

2. Put all ingredients to your bread machine (except olives), carefully following the instructions of the manufacturer.

3. Set the program of your bread machine to French bread and set crust type to Medium.

4. Once the maker beeps, add olives.

5. Wait until the cycle completes.

6. Once the loaf is ready, take the bucket out and cool the loaf for 6 minutes.

7. Wobble the bucket to take off the loaf.

Nutrition:

Total Carbs: 71g

Fiber: 1g

Protein: 10g

Fat: 7g

Calories: 386

13.   Lovely Aromatic Lavender Bread

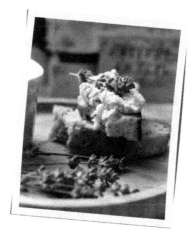

Preparation Time: 5 minutes

Cooking Time: 2 hours and 45 minutes

Servings: 8 slices

Ingredients:

- ¾ cup milk at 80 degrees F

- 1 tablespoon melted butter, cooled

- 1 tablespoon sugar

- ¾ teaspoon salt

- 1 teaspoon fresh lavender flower, chopped

- ¼ teaspoon lemon zest

- ¼ teaspoon fresh thyme, chopped

- 2 cups white bread flour

- ¾ teaspoon instant yeast

Directions:

1. Add all of the ingredients to your bread machine, carefully following the instructions of the manufacturer.

2. Set the program of your bread machine to Basic/White Bread and set crust type to Medium.

3. Wait until the cycle completes.

4. Once the loaf is ready, take the bucket out and let the loaf cool for 5 minutes.

5. Gently shake the bucket to remove the loaf.

Nutrition:

Total Carbs: 27g

Fiber: 1g

Protein: 4g

Fat: 2g

Calories: 144

CHAPTER 8:

Rolls and Pizza

14.   Sweet Potato Rolls

Preparation Time: 25 Minutes

Cooking Time: 40 Minutes

Servings: 8

Ingredients:

- Two meshed medium sweet potatoes
- 1 cup milk
- 3.2 tablespoons melted butter
- 1 large beaten egg
- 4 cups all-purpose flour
- 4 tablespoons sugar
- 1 teaspoon salt
- 2.5 teaspoons active dry yeast

Directions:

1. Peel potatoes and cut in cubes
2. Boil salted water

3. Add potato to water and reduce the heat. Cover the pan and cook for about 22 minutes

4. Drain and mash

5. Cool and measure 1 cup

6. Add Ingredients to the bread machine according to manufacturer's recommendations

7. Use the basic dough cycle

8. When it finishes, tear pieces to make balls, place in a baking pan

9. Cover rolls through a cloth and let rise for about 40 minutes

10. Preheat oven to 370 F

11. Bake until nicely browned

12. Brush the tops with melted or softened butter

Nutrition:

Carbs – 28 G

Fat – 3 G

Protein – 6 G

Calories – 160

15.   Cinnamon Rolls

Preparation Time: 5 Minutes

Cooking Time: 25 Minutes

Servings: 8

Ingredients:

- 1 cup milk
- 1 large egg
- tablespoons butter
    - cups bread flour
    - tablespoons sugar
- 0.5 teaspoon salt
    - teaspoons active dry yeast
- 0.5 cup butter
- 0.5 cup sugar
- teaspoons cinnamon
- 0.5 teaspoon nutmeg
- 0.3 cup nuts
- 1 cup of powdered sugar
- tablespoons milk
- 0.5 teaspoon vanilla

Directions:

Cinnamon Rolls:

1. Add ingredients for the cinnamon rolls to bread machine according to manufacturer's recommendations

2. Use dough cycle

3. Place dough onto a floured surface when the cycle is done

4. Knead the dough for one minute, let it rest for 15 minutes

5. Preheat oven to 370 F

6. Roll the dough out in a rectangle

7. Spread melted butter over the dough

8. Sprinkle sugar, cinnamon, nutmeg, chopped nuts

9. Roll the dough up on the side

10. Press edges and form into evenly shaped roll

11. Cut the entire roll into one-inch pieces

12. Place rolls into a baking pan

13. Cover and let the dough and wait for it to rise until double in size

14. This part will take 30 to 45 minutes

15. Bake the rolls until golden brown

16. Cool in pan for 15 minutes, drizzle with powdered sugar icing

Icing:

1. Combine powdered sugar, milk, vanilla

2. Blend until smooth

Nutrition:

Carbs – 28 G

Fat – 3 G

Protein – 6 G Calories – 160

16.   Blueberry Rolls

Preparation Time: 50 Minutes

Cooking Time: 25 - 40 Minutes

Servings: 8

Ingredients:

- 1 cup milk

- 1 large egg

- 2 teaspoons vanilla extract

- 3 cups all-purpose flour

- 0.3 cup sugar

- 1.2 teaspoon salt

- 2 tablespoons butter

- 1 tablespoon active dry yeast

- 1.2 cup blueberries

- 1.2 teaspoon cinnamon

- 1 tablespoon water

- 1 large egg yolk

For the Vanilla Icing:

- 4 cups confectioners' sugar

- 1 tablespoon butter

- 1 teaspoon vanilla extract

- 2 tablespoons water

Directions:

1. Whisk milk with egg and vanilla extract

2. Add milk flour mixture, sugar, salt, butter and yeast to the bread machine pan according to manufacturer's recommendations

3. Start on the dough cycle

4. Add blueberries and ground cinnamon at beep

5. Grease a baking pan

6. Put dough onto a floured surface and punch it

7. Knead, adding more flour, if needed

8. Shape the dough into balls and place them in the prepared round pan

9. Cover the pan with a kitchen towel and let the rolls rise for 40 minutes

10. Heat the oven to 355 F

11. Whisk water and egg yolk

12. Brush the mixture over the rolls

13. Bake for 25 minutes

14. Remove to a rack and let cool

Icing:

15. Combine sugar with melted butter and vanilla extract

16. Add hot water

17. Transfer the rolls to a rack

18. Drizzle the icing over the rolls

Nutrition:

Carbs – 28 G Fat – 3 GProtein – 6 G Calories – 160

17.   Mini Maple Cinnamon Rolls

Preparation Time: 25 - 30 Minutes

Cooking Time: 25 Minutes

Servings: 12

Ingredients:

- 2 cup whole milk
- 1.2 cup maple syrup
- 1.2 cup butter
- 1 large egg
- 1 teaspoon salt
- 3 cups bread flour
- 0.5 ounces active dry yeast
- 0.5 cup packed brown sugar
- 2 tablespoons bread flour
- 4 teaspoons ground cinnamon
- 2 tablespoons cold butter

Directions:

1. Select dough setting
2. When the cycle completes, turn dough onto a floured surface
3. Roll into two rectangles
4. Combine brown sugar, flour, cinnamon
5. Cut in butter
6. Sprinkle half over rectangles

7. Roll up, pinch seam to seal

8. Cut each into 12 slices

9. Place in a baking pan

10. Cover and let rise for 20 minutes

11. Bake at 370° F until golden brown

12. Cool for 5 minutes

13. Combine butter, confectioners' sugar, syrup and milk

14. Spread over rolls

Nutrition:

Carbs – 28 G

Fat – 3 G

Protein – 6 G

Calories – 160

r

CHAPTER 9:

Classic Breads

18.   Almond Flour Bread

Preparation Time: 10 Minutes

Cooking Time: 10 Minutes

Servings: 10

Ingredients:

- Four egg whites
- Two egg yolks
- 2 cups almond flour
- 1/4 cup butter, melted
- 2 tbsp. psyllium husk powder
- 1 1/2 tbsp. baking powder
- 1/2 tsp. xanthan gum
- Salt
- 1/2 cup + 2 tbsp. warm water
- 2 1/4 tsp. yeast

Directions:

1. Make use of a small mixing bowl to combine the dry ingredients except for the yeast.

2. In the bread machine pan, add all the wet ingredients.

3. Add all of your dry ingredients from the lower mixing bowl to the bread machine pan. Top with the yeast.

4. Set the bread machine to the basic bread setting.

5. When the bread is completed, remove the bread machine pan from the bread machine.

6. Let cool a little before moving to a cooling rack.

7. The bread can be stored for up to 4 days on the counter and three months in the freezer.

Nutrition:

Calories: 110

Carbohydrates: 2.4g

Protein: 4g

Fat: 10g

19.   Coconut Flour Bread

Preparation Time: 10 Minutes

Cooking Time: 15 Minutes

Servings: 12

Ingredients:

- Six eggs
- 1/2 cup coconut flour
- 2 tbsp. psyllium husk
- 1/4 cup olive oil
- 1 1/2 tsp. salt
- 1 tbsp. xanthan gum
- 1 tbsp. baking powder
- 2 1/4 tsp. yeast

Directions:

1. Use a small mixing bowl to combine dry ingredients except for the yeast.

2. In the bread machine pan, add all the wet ingredients.

3. Add all of your dry ingredients from the small mixing bowl to the bread machine pan. Top with the yeast.

4. Set the bread machine to the basic bread setting.

5. When the bread is done, eradicate the bread machine pan from the bread machine.

6. Let cool slightly before transferring to a cooling rack.

7. The bread can be stockpiled for up to 4 days on the counter and three months in the freezer.

Nutrition:

Calories: 174

Carbohydrates: 4g

Protein: 7g

Fat: 15g

20.   Cloud Bread Loaf

Preparation Time: 10 Minutes

Cooking Time: 15 Minutes

Servings: 10

Ingredients:

- Six egg whites
- Six egg yolks
- 1/2 cup whey protein powder, unflavored
- 1/2 tsp. cream of tartar
- 6 oz. sour cream
- 1/2 tsp. baking powder
- 1/4 tsp. garlic powder
- 1/4 tsp. onion powder
- 1/4 tsp. salt

Directions:

1. Beat the egg whites, including the cream of tartar, till you have stiff peaks forming. Set aside.
2. Combine all other ingredients into another bowl and mix.
3. Fold the mixtures together, a little at a time.
4. Pour mixture into your bread machine pan.
5. Set the bread machine to quick bread.
6. When the bread is finished, remove the bread machine pan from the bread machine.

7. Let cool slightly before transferring to a cooling bracket.

8. The bread may be kept for up to 3 days on the counter.

Nutrition:

Calories: 90

Carbohydrates: 2g

Protein: 6g

Fat: 7g

21.   Sandwich Buns

Preparation Time: 10 Minutes

Cooking Time: 25 Minutes

Servings: 8

Ingredients:

- Four eggs
- 2 ½ oz. almond flour
- 1 Tbsp. coconut flour
- 1 oz. psyllium
- 1 ½ cups eggplant, finely grated, juices drained
- 3 Tbsp. sesame seeds
- 1 ½ tsp. baking powder
- Salt to taste

Directions:

1. Whisk eggs until foamy, and then add grated eggplant.
2. In a separate bowl, mix all dry ingredients.
3. Add them to the egg mixture. Mix well.
4. Line a baking sheet with parchment paper, then shape the buns with your hands.
5. Bake at 374F for 20 to 25 minutes.

Nutrition:

Calories: 99 Fat: 6g Carb: 10g

Protein: 5.3g

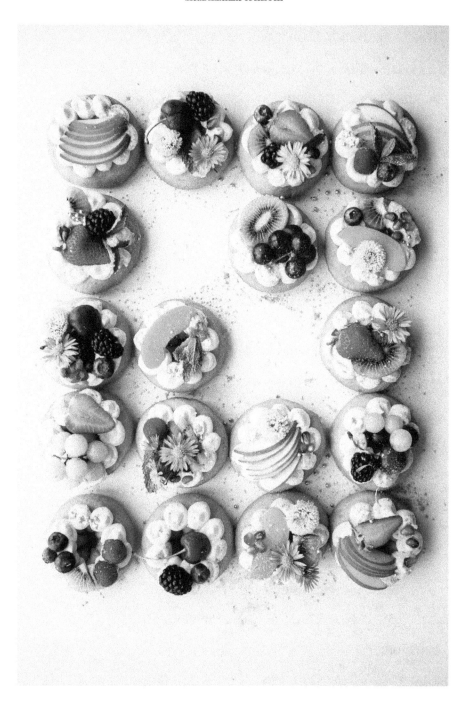

CHAPTER 10:

Nut and Seed Breads

22.   Flax and Sunflower Seed Bread

Preparation Time: 5 Minutes

Cooking Time: 25 Minutes

Servings: 8

Ingredients:

- 1 1/3 cups water
- Two tablespoons butter softened
- Three tablespoons honey
- 2/3 cups of bread flour
- One teaspoon salt
- One teaspoon active dry yeast
- 1/2 cup flax seeds
- 1/2 cup sunflower seeds

Directions:

1. With the manufacturer's suggested order, add all the ingredients (apart from sunflower seeds) to the bread machine's pan.

2. The select basic white cycle, then press start.

3. Just in the knead cycle that your machine signals alert sounds, add the sunflower seeds.

Nutrition:

Calories: 140 calories;

Sodium: 169

Total Carbohydrate: 22.7

Cholesterol: 4

Protein: 4.2 Total Fat: 4.2

23. Honey and Flaxseed Bread

Preparation Time: 5 Minutes

Cooking Time: 25 Minutes

Servings: 8

Ingredients:

- 1 1/8 cups water
- 1 1/2 tablespoons flaxseed oil
- Three tablespoons honey
- 1/2 tablespoon liquid lecithin
- cups whole wheat flour
- 1/2 cup flax seed
- Two tablespoons bread flour
- Three tablespoons whey powder
- 1 1/2 teaspoons sea salt
- Two teaspoons active dry yeast

Directions:

1. In the bread machine pan, put in all of the ingredients following the order recommended by the manufacturer.
2. Choose the Wheat cycle on the machine and press the Start button to run the machine.

Nutrition:

Calories: 174 calories; Protein: 7.1 Total Fat: 4.9

Sodium: 242 Total Carbohydrate: 30.8

Cholesterol: 1

24.   Pumpkin and Sunflower Seed Bread

Preparation Time: 5 Minutes

Cooking Time: 25 Minutes

Servings: 8

Ingredients:

- 1 (.25 ounce) package instant yeast
- 1 cup of warm water
- 1/4 cup honey
- Four teaspoons vegetable oil
- cups whole wheat flour
- 1/4 cup wheat bran (optional)
- One teaspoon salt
- 1/3 cup sunflower seeds
- 1/3 cup shelled, toasted, chopped pumpkin seeds

Directions:

1 Into the bread machine, put the ingredients according to the order suggested by the manufacturer.

2 Next is setting the machine to the whole wheat setting, then press the start button.

3 You can add the pumpkin and sunflower seeds at the beep if your bread machine has a signal for nuts or fruit.

Nutrition: Calories: 148 calories; Total Carbohydrate: 24.1

Cholesterol: 0 Protein: 5.1 Total Fat: 4.8

Sodium: 158

25.   Seven Grain Bread

Preparation Time: 5 Minutes

Cooking Time: 25 Minutes

Servings: 8

Ingredients:

- 1 1/3 cups warm water
- One tablespoon active dry yeast
- Three tablespoons dry milk powder
- Two tablespoons vegetable oil
- Two tablespoons honey
- Two teaspoons salt
- One egg
- 1 cup whole wheat flour
- 1/2 cups bread flour
- 3/4 cup 7-grain cereal

Directions:

1   Follow the order of putting the ingredients into the pan of the bread machine recommended by the manufacturer.

2   Choose the Whole Wheat Bread cycle on the machine and press the Start button to run the machine.

Nutrition:

Calories: 285 calories; Total Fat: 5.2

Sodium: 629 Total Carbohydrate: 50.6

Cholesterol: 24 Protein: 9.8

CHAPTER 11:

Grain, Seed & Nut Bread

26. Sunflower & Flax Seed Bread

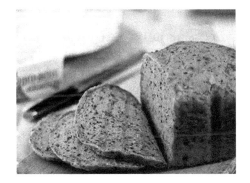

Preparation Time: 5 minutes

Cooking Time: 3 hours

Servings: 10 slices

Ingredients:

- Water – 1 1/3 cups.

- Butter – 2 tablespoons.

- Honey – 3 tablespoons.

- Bread flour – 1 ½ cups.

- Whole wheat flour – 1 1/3 cups.

- Salt – 1 teaspoon.

- Active dry yeast – 1 teaspoon.

- Flax seeds – ½ cup.

- Sunflower seeds – ½ cup.

Directions:

1. Add all ingredients except for sunflower seeds into the bread machine pan.

2. Select basic setting then select light/medium crust and press start.

3. Add sunflower seeds just before the final kneading cycle.

4. Once loaf is done, remove the loaf pan from the machine. Allow it to cool for 10 minutes. Slice and serve.

Nutrition: Calories 220, Carbs 36.6g, Fat 5.7g,

Protein 6.6g

27.   Nutritious 9-Grain Bread

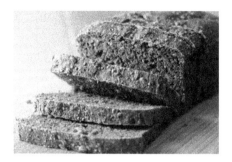

Preparation Time: 5 minutes

Cooking Time: 2 hours

Servings: 10 slices

Ingredients:

- Warm water – 3/4 cup+2 tablespoons.

- Whole wheat flour – 1 cup.

- Bread flour – 1 cup.

- 9-grain cereal – ½ cup., crushed

- Salt – 1 teaspoon.

- Butter – 1 tablespoon.

- Sugar – 2 tablespoons.

- Milk powder – 1 tablespoon.

- Active dry yeast – 2 teaspoons.

Directions:

1. Put all ingredients into the bread machine.

2. Select whole wheat setting then select light/medium crust and start.

3. Once loaf is done, remove the loaf pan from the machine.

4. Allow it to cool for 10 minutes. Slice and serve.

Nutrition:

Calories 132, Carbs 25g,

Fat 1.7g, Protein 4.1g

CHAPTER 12:

Fruit and Vegetable Bread

28. Sun Vegetable Bread

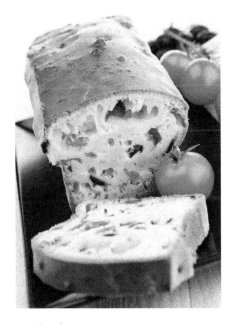

Preparation Time: 15 minutes

Cooking Time: 3 hours 45 minutes

Servings: 8 slices

Ingredients:

- 2 cups (250 g) wheat flour

- 2 cups (250 g) whole-wheat flour

- 2 teaspoons panifarin
- 2 teaspoons yeast
- 1½ teaspoons salt
- 1 tablespoon sugar
- 1 tablespoon paprika dried slices
- 2 tablespoons dried beets
- 1 tablespoon dried garlic
- 1½ cups water
- 1 tablespoon vegetable oil

Directions:

1. Set baking program, which should be 4 hours; crust color is Medium.
2. Be sure to look at the kneading phase of the dough, to get a smooth and soft bun.

Nutrition:

Calories 253; Total Fat 2.6g;

Saturated Fat 0.5g; Cholesterol 0g;

Sodium 444mg; Total Carbohydrate 49.6g;

Dietary Fiber 2.6g; Total Sugars 0.6g;

Protein 7.2g

29.   Tomato Onion Bread

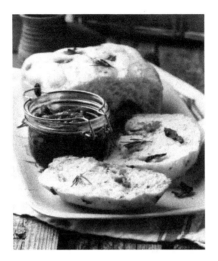

Preparation Time: 10 minutes

Cooking Time: 3 hours 50 minutes

Servings: 12 slices

Ingredients:

- 2 cups all-purpose flour

- 1 cup whole meal flour

- ½ cup warm water

- 4 3/4 ounces (140 ml) milk

- 3 tablespoons olive oil

- 2 tablespoons sugar

- 1 teaspoon salt

- 2 teaspoons dry yeast

- ½ teaspoon baking powder

- 5 sun-dried tomatoes

- 1 onion

- ¼ teaspoon black pepper

Directions:

1. Prepare all the necessary products. Finely chop the onion and sauté in a frying pan. Cut up the sun-dried tomatoes (10 halves).

2. Pour all liquid ingredients into the bowl; then cover with flour and put in the tomatoes and onions. Pour in the yeast and baking powder, without touching the liquid.

3. Select the baking mode and start. You can choose the Bread with Additives program, and then the bread maker will knead the dough at low speeds.

Nutrition:

Calories 241; Total Fat 6.4g;

Saturated Fat 1.1g; Cholesterol 1g;

Sodium 305mg; Total Carbohydrate 40g;

Dietary Fiber 3.5g; Total Sugars 6.8g;

Protein 6.7g

30. Tomato Bread

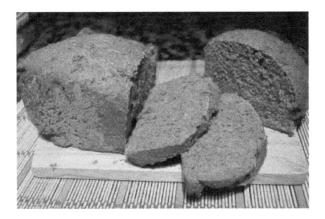

Preparation Time: 5 minutes **Cooking Time:** 3 hours 30 minutes**Servings:** 8 slices

Ingredients:

- 3 tablespoons tomato paste
- 1½ cups (340 ml) water
- 4 1/3 cups (560 g) flour
- 1½ tablespoon vegetable oil
- 2 teaspoons sugar
- 2 teaspoons salt
- 1 ½ teaspoons dry yeast
- ½ teaspoon oregano, dried
- ½ teaspoon ground sweet paprika

Directions:

1. Dilute the tomato paste in warm water. If you do not like the tomato flavor, reduce the amount of tomato paste, but putting

less than 1 tablespoon does not make sense, because the color will fade.

2. Prepare the spices. I added a little more oregano as well as Provencal herbs to the oregano and paprika (this bread also begs for spices).

3. Sieve the flour to enrich it with oxygen. Add the spices to the flour and mix well.

4. Pour the vegetable oil into the bread maker container. Add the tomato/water mixture, sugar, salt, and then the flour with spices, and then the yeast.

5. Turn on the bread maker (the Basic program – I have the WHITE BREAD – the crust Medium).

6. After the end of the baking cycle, turn off the bread maker. Remove the bread container and take out the hot bread. Place it on the grate for cooling for 1 hour.

Nutrition:

Calories 281; Total Fat 3.3g; Saturated Fat 0.6g;

Cholesterol 0g; Sodium 590mg; Total Carbohydrate 54.3g; ietary Fiber 2.4g;

Total Sugars 1.9g;

Protein 7.6g

CHAPTER 13:

Holiday Bread

31.   Pumpkin Bread

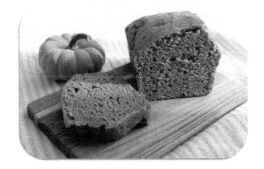

Preparation time: 5 minutes

Cooking time: 1 hour

Servings: 14

Ingredients:

- ½ cup plus 2 tablespoons warm water

- ½ cup canned pumpkin puree

- ¼ cup butter, softened

- ¼ cup non-fat dry milk powder

- 2¾ cups bread flour

- ¼ cup brown sugar

- ¾ teaspoon salt

- 1 teaspoon ground cinnamon

- ½ teaspoon ground ginger

- 1/8 teaspoon ground nutmeg

- 2¼ teaspoons active dry yeast

Directions:

1. Place all ingredients in the baking pan of the bread machine in the order recommended by the manufacturer.

2. Place the baking pan in the bread machine and close the lid.

3. Select Basic setting.

4. Press the start button.

5. Carefully, remove the baking pan from the machine and then invert the bread loaf onto a wire rack to cool completely before slicing.

6. With a sharp knife, cut bread loaf into desired-sized slices and serve.

Nutrition:

Calories 134 Total Fat 3.6 g

Saturated Fat 2.1 g Cholesterol 9 mg

Sodium 149 mg

Total Carbs 22.4 g

Fiber 1.1 g

Sugar 2.9 g

Protein 2.9 g

32.   Pumpkin Cranberry Bread

Preparation time: 10 minutes

Cooking time: 4 hours

Servings: 12

Ingredients:

- ¾ cup water

- 2/3 cup canned pumpkin

- 3 tablespoons brown sugar

- 2 tablespoons vegetable oil

- 2 cups all-purpose flour

- 1 cup whole-wheat flour

- 1¼ teaspoon salt

- ½ cup sweetened dried cranberries

- ½ cup walnuts, chopped

- 1¾ teaspoons active dry yeast

Directions:

1. Place all ingredients in the baking pan of the bread machine in the order recommended by the manufacturer.

2. Place the baking pan in the bread machine and close the lid.

3. Select Basic setting.

4. Press the start button.

5. Carefully, remove the baking pan from the machine and then invert the bread loaf onto a wire rack to cool completely before slicing.

6. With a sharp knife, cut bread loaf into desired-sized slices and serve.

Nutrition:

Calories 199

Total Fat 6 g

Saturated Fat 0.7 g

Cholesterol 0 mg

Sodium 247 mg

Total Carbs 31.4 g

Fiber 3.2 g

Sugar 5.1 g

Protein 5.6 g

CHAPTER 14:

Sweet Breads

33.   Brownie Bread

Preparation Time: 1 hour 15 minutes

Cooking Time: 50 minutes

Servings: 1 loaf

Ingredients:

- 1 egg
- 1 egg yolk
- 1 teaspoon Salt
- 1/2 cup boiling water
- 1/2 cup cocoa powder, unsweetened
- 1/2 cup warm water
- 1/2 teaspoon Active dry yeast
- tablespoon Vegetable oil
- teaspoon White sugar
- 2/3 cup white sugar
- cups bread flour

Directions:

1 Put the cocoa powder in a small bow. Pour boiling water and dissolve the cocoa powder.

2 Put the warm water, yeast and the 2 teaspoon White sugar in another bowl. Dissolve yeast and sugar. Let stand for about 10 minutes, or until the mix is creamy.

3 Place the cocoa mix, the yeast mix, the flour, the 2/3 cup white sugar, the salt, the vegetable, and the egg in the bread pan. Select basic bread cycle. Press start.

Nutrition:

Calories: 70 Cal

Fat   : 3 g

Carbohydrates: 10 g

Protein : 1 g

34.   Black Forest Bread

Preparation Time: 2 hour 15 minutes

Cooking Time: 50 minutes

Servings: 1 loaf

Ingredients:

- 1 1/8 cups Warm water
- 1/3 cup Molasses
- 1 1/2 tablespoons Canola oil
- 1 1/2 cups Bread flour
- 1 cup Rye flour
- 1 cup Whole wheat flour
- 1 1/2 teaspoons Salt
- tablespoons Cocoa powder
- 1 1/2 tablespoons Caraway seeds
- teaspoons Active dry yeast

Directions:

1   Place all ingredients into your bread maker according to manufacture.

2   Select type to a light crust.

3   Press start.

4   Remembering to check while starting to knead.

5   If mixture is too dry add tablespoon warm water at a time.

6   If mixture is too wet add flour again a little at a time.

7   Mixture should go into a ball form, and just soft and slightly sticky to the finger touch. This goes for all types of breads when kneading.

Nutrition:

Calories: 240 Cal

Fat   : 4 g

Carbohydrates: 29 g

Protein : 22 g

35. Sweet Almond Anise Bread

Preparation Time: 2 hours 20 minutes

Cooking Time: 50 minutes

Servings: 1 loaf

Ingredients:

- ¾ cup water
- ¼ cup butter
- ¼ cup sugar
- ½ teaspoon salt
- cups bread flour
- 1 teaspoon anise seed
- teaspoons active dry yeast
- ½ cup almonds, chopped

Directions:

1 Add all of the ingredients to your bread machine, carefully following the instructions of the manufacturer
2 Set the program of your bread machine to Basic/White Bread and set crust type to Medium
3 Press START
4 Wait until the cycle completes
5 Once the loaf is ready, take the bucket out and let the loaf cool for 5 minutes
6 Gently shake the bucket to remove the loaf
7 Transfer to a cooling rack, slice and serve

8 Enjoy!

Nutrition:

Calories: 87 Cal

Fat: 4 g

Carbohydrates: 7 g

Protein : 3 g

Fiber: 1 g

36. Chocolate Ginger and Hazelnut Bread

Preparation Time: 2 hours 50 minutes

Cooking Time: 45 minutes

Servings: 2 loaves

Ingredients:

- 1/2 cup chopped hazelnuts
- teaspoon bread machine yeast
- 1/2 cups bread flour
- 1 teaspoon salt
- 1 1/2 tablespoon dry skim milk powder
- tablespoon light brown sugar
- tablespoon candied ginger, chopped
- 1/3 cup unsweetened coconut
- 1 1/2 tablespoon unsalted butter, cubed
- 1 cup, plus 2 tablespoon water, with a temperature of 80 to 90 degrees F (26 to 32 degrees C)

Directions:

1 Put all the ingredients, except the hazelnuts, in the pan in this order: water, butter, coconut, candied ginger, brown sugar, milk, salt, flour, and yeast.

2 Secure the pan in the machine and close the lid. Put the toasted hazelnuts in the fruit and nut dispenser.

3 Turn the machine on. Select the basic setting and your desired color of the crust and press start.

4 Once done, carefully transfer the baked bread to a wire rack until cooled.

Nutrition:

Calories: 273 calories;

Total Carbohydrate: 43 g

Total Fat: 11 g

Protein: 7 g

37. White Chocolate Bread

Preparation 3 hours **Cooking :** 15 minutes **Servings:** 12

Ingredients:

- 1/4 cup warm water
- 1 cup warm milk
- 1 egg
- 1/4 cup butter, softened
- cups bread flour
- tablespoons brown sugar
- tablespoons white sugar
- 1 teaspoon salt
- 1 teaspoon ground cinnamon
- 1 (.25 oz.) package active dry yeast
- 1 cup white chocolate chips

Directions:

1 Put all the ingredients together, except for the white chocolate chips, into the bread machine pan following the order suggested by the manufacturer. Choose the cycle on the machine and press the Start button to run the machine. Put in the white chocolate chips at the machine's signal if the machine used has a Fruit setting on it or you may put the white chocolate chips about 5 minutes before the kneading cycle ends.

Nutrition: Calories: 277 calories; Total Carbohydrate: 39 g Cholesterol: 30 mg Total Fat: 10.5 g Protein: 6.6 gSodium: 253 mg

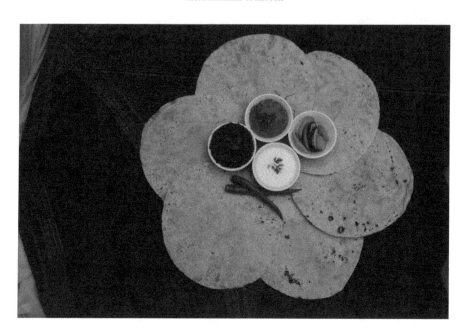

CHAPTER 15:

SourdoughErrore. Il segnalibro non è definito. Breads

38.   Honey Sourdough Bread

Preparation Time: 15 minutes 1 week (Starter)

Cooking Time: 3 hours

Servings: 1 loaf

Ingredients:

- 2/3 cup sourdough starter
- 1/2 cup water
- 1 tablespoon vegetable oil
- 2 tablespoons honey
- 1/2 teaspoon salt
- 1/2 cup high protein wheat flour
- 2 cups bread flour
- 1 teaspoon active dry yeast

Directions:

1. Measure 1 cup of starter and remaining bread ingredients, add to bread machine pan.

2. Choose basic/white bread cycle with medium or light crust color.

Nutrition:

Calories: 175 calories; Total Carbohydrate: 33 g

Total Fat: 0.3 g Protein: 5.6 g

Sodium: 121 mg Fiber: 1.9 g

CHAPTER 16:

Cheese Breads

39.   Cheddar Cheese Basil Bread

Preparation Time: 10 Minutes

Cooking Time: 25 Minutes

Servings: 8

Ingredients:

- 1 cup milk
- One tablespoon melted butter cooled
- One tablespoon sugar
- One teaspoon dried basil
- ¾ cup (3 ounces) shredded sharp Cheddar cheese
- ¾ teaspoon salt
- cups white bread flour
- 1½ teaspoons active dry yeast

Directions:

1   Preparing the Ingredients. Place the ingredients in your Zojirushi bread machine.

2   Select the Bake cycle. Program the machine for Regular Basic, choose light or medium crust, and then press Start.

3   If the loaf is done, remove the bucket from the machine.

4   Let the loaf cool for 5 minutes.

5   Softly shake the canister to remove the loaf and put it out onto a rack to cool.

Nutrition:

Calories 174 Carbs 31.1g Fat 3.1g Protein 5.1g

40. Herb and Parmesan Cheese Loaf

Cooking Time: 25 Minutes Preparation Time: 10 Minutes

Servings: 8

Ingredients:

- cups + 2 tbsp. all-purpose flour
- 1 cup of water
- tbsp. oil
- tbsp. sugar
- tbsp. milk
- 1 tbsp. instant yeast
- 1 tsp. garlic powder
- tbsp. parmesan cheese
- 1 tbsp. fresh basil
- 1 tbsp. fresh oregano
- 1 tbsp. fresh chives or rosemary

Directions:

1 Preparing the Ingredients. Place all fixings in the bread pan in the liquid-cheese and herb-dry-yeast layering.
2 Put the pan in the Zojirushi bread machine.
3 Select the Bake cycle. Choose Regular Basic Setting.
4 Press start and wait until the loaf is cooked.
5 The machine will start the keep warm mode after the bread is complete.

6   Just allow it to stay in that mode for about 10 minutes before unplugging.

7   Remove the pan and wait for it to cool down for about 10 minutes.

Nutrition:

Calories 174 Carbs 31.1g

Fat 3.1g Protein 5.1g

CHAPTER 17:

Keto Bread Recipes

41.   Toast Bread

Preparation Time: 3 ½ hours **Cooking Time:** 3 ½ hours

Servings: 8

Ingredients:

- 1 ½ teaspoons yeast
- cups almond flour
- tablespoons sugar
- 1 teaspoon salt
- 1 ½ tablespoon butter
- 1 cup water

Directions:

1   Pour water into the bowl; add salt, sugar, soft butter, flour, and yeast.

2   I add dried tomatoes and paprika.

3   Put it on the basic program.

4   The crust can be light or medium.

Nutrition: carbohydrates 5 g fats 2.7 g protein 5.2 g calories 203 fiber 1 g

42.   Walnut Bread

Preparation Time: 4 hours

Cooking Time: 4 hours

Servings: 10

Ingredients:

- cups almond flour
- ½ cup water
- ½ cup milk
- eggs
- ½ cup walnuts
- 1 tablespoon vegetable oil
- 1 tablespoon sugar
- 1 teaspoon salt
- 1 teaspoon yeast

Directions

1   All products must be room temperature.

2   Pour water, milk, and vegetable oil into the bucket and add in the eggs.

3   Now pour in the sifted almond flour. In the process of kneading bread, you may need a little more or less flour – it depends on its moisture.

4   Pour in salt, sugar, and yeast. If it is hot in the kitchen (especially in summer), pour all three Ingredients into the different ends of the bucket so that the dough does not have time for peroxide.

5   Now the first kneading dough begins, which lasts 15 minutes. In the process, we monitor the state of the ball. It should be soft, but at the same time, keep its shape and not spread. If the ball does not want to be collected, add a little flour, since the moisture of this product is different for everyone. If the bucket is clean and all the flour is incorporated into the dough, then everything is done right. If the dough is still lumpy and even crumbles, you need to add a little more liquid.

6   Close the lid and then prepare the nuts. They need to be sorted and lightly fried in a dry frying pan; the pieces of nuts will be crispy. Then let them cool and cut with a knife to the desired size. When the bread maker signals, pour in the nuts and wait until the spatula mixes them into the dough.

7   Remove the bucket and take out the walnut bread. Completely cool it on a grill so that the bottom does not get wet.

Nutrition: carbohydrates 4 g fats 6.7 g protein 8.3 g calories 257 fiber 1.3 g

43.   Bulgur Bread

Preparation Time: 3 hours **Cooking Time:** 3 hours

Servings: 8

Ingredients:

- ½ cup bulgur
- 1/3 cup boiling water
- 1 egg
- 1 cup water
- 1 tablespoon butter
- 1 ½ tablespoon milk powder
- 1 tablespoon sugar
- teaspoons salt
- ¼ cups flour
- 1 teaspoon dried yeast

Directions:

1   Bulgur pour boiling water into a small container and cover with a lid. Leave to stand for 30 minutes.

2   Cut butter into small cubes.

3   Stir the egg with water in a measuring container. The total volume of eggs with water should be 300 ml.

4   Put all the Ingredients in the bread maker in the order that is described in the instructions for your bread maker. Bake in the basic mode, medium crust.

Nutrition: carbohydrates 3 g fats 3 g protein 8.9 g calories 255 fiber 1.2 g

44.   Italian Blue Cheese Bread

Preparation Time: 3 hours

Cooking Time: 3 hours

Servings: 8

Ingredients:

- 1 teaspoon dry yeast
- ½ cups almond flour
- 1 ½ teaspoon salt
- 1 tablespoon sugar
- 1 tablespoon olive oil
- ½ cup blue cheese
- 1 cup water

Directions

1   Mix all the Ingredients. Start baking.

Nutrition: carbohydrates 5 g fats 4.6 g protein 6 g calories 194 fiber 1.5 g

45.   Milk Almond Bread

Preparation Time: 3 ½ hours

Cooking Time: 3 ½ hours

Servings: 8

Ingredients:

- 1 ¼ cup milk
- ¼ cups almond flour
- tablespoons butter
- teaspoons dry yeast
- 1 tablespoon sugar
- teaspoons salt

Directions

1 Pour the milk into the form and ½ cup of water. Add flour.

2 Put butter, sugar, and salt in different corners of the mold. Make a groove in the flour and put in the yeast.

3 Bake on the basic program.

4 Cool the bread.

Nutrition: carbohydrates 5 g fats 4.5 g protein 10.1 g calories 352 fiber 1.5 g

46. Zucchini bread

Preparation Time: 2 hours 10 minutes

Cooking Time: 2 hours 10 minutes

Servings: 8

Ingredients:

- whole eggs
- ¼ teaspoon sea salt
- 1 cup olive oil
- 1 cup white sugar
- 1 tablespoon vanilla sugar
- teaspoon cinnamon
- ½ cup nuts, ground
- cups bread flour, well sifted
- 1 tablespoon baking powder
- 1¼ cup zucchini, grated

Directions:

1   Prepare all of the ingredients for your bread and measuring means (a cup, a spoon, kitchen scales).

2   Carefully measure the ingredients into the pan, except the zucchini and nuts.

3   Place all of the ingredients into the bread bucket in the right order, following the manual for your bread machine.

4   Close the cover.

5   Select the program of your bread machine to CAKE and choose the crust color to LIGHT.

6 Press START.

7 After the signal, put the grated zucchini and nuts to the dough.

8 Wait until the program completes.

9 When done, take the bucket out and let it cool for 5-10 minutes.

10 Shake the loaf from the pan and let cool for 30 minutes on a cooling rack.

11 Slice, serve, and enjoy the taste of fragrant homemade bread.

Nutrition:

Carbohydrates 4 g

Fats 31 g

Protein 8.6 g

Calories 556

Fiber 1.3 g

47.   Macadamia Nut Bread

Preparation Time: 5 minutes

Cooking Time: 21 min

Serving: 6

Ingredients:

- oz. macadamia nuts I utilized the Royal Hawaiian brand
- enormous eggs
- 1/4 cup coconut flour (28 g)
- 1/2 teaspoon heating pop
- 1/2 teaspoon apple juice vinegar

Direction:

1   Preheat broiler to 350F.

2   To a blender or nourishment processor, include macadamia nuts and heartbeat until it becomes nut margarine. On the off chance that your blender doesn't work superbly without fluid, include eggs each in turn until the consistency is that of a nut margarine.

3   Scrape drawbacks of blender or nourishment processor, and include remaining eggs. Mix until well-fused.

4   Add in coconut flour, heating pop, and apple juice vinegar and heartbeat until consolidated.

5   Grease a standard-size bread dish and include hitter. Smooth surface of hitter and spot-on a base rack of the broiler for 30-40 minutes, or until the top is brilliant dark-colored.

6   Remove from stove and permit to cool in prospect 20 minutes before evacuating.

7　Will store in a water/air proof compartment at room temperature for 3-4 days at room temperature or for multi-week in the refrigerator

Nutrition:

Cal: 40,

Carbs: 4g

Net Carbs: 3.5 g,

Fiber: 8.5 g,

Fat: 14 g,

Protein: 10g,

Sugars: 3 g.

Sugars: 3 g.

48.   Buttery & Soft Skillet Flatbread

Preparation Time: 9 minutes

Cooking Time: 22 min

Servings: 8

Ingredients:

- 1 cup Almond Flour
- teaspoon Coconut Flour
- teaspoon Xanthan Gum
- 1/2 teaspoon heating Powder
- 1/2 teaspoon Falk Salt
- 1 Whole Egg + 1 Egg White
- 1 teaspoon Water
- 1 teaspoon Oil for searing
- 1 teaspoon liquefied Butter-for slathering

Directions:

1   Whisk together the dry fixings (flours, thickener, preparing powder, salt) until very much consolidated.

2   Add the egg and egg white and beat tenderly into the flour to fuse. The mixture will start to frame.

3   Add the tablespoon of water and start to work the batter to permit the flour and thickener to retain the dampness.

4   Cut the batter in 4 equivalent parts and press each area out with stick wrap. Watch the video for directions!

5   Heat a huge skillet over medium warmth and include oil.

6   Fry every flatbread for around 1 min on each side.

7   Brush with margarine (while hot) and embellish with salt and cleaved parsley.

Nutrition:

Cal: 50,

Carbs: 10g/

Net Carbs: 6g,

Fiber: 4.5 g,

Fat: 8 g,

Protein: 9g,

Sugars: 3 g.

49. Cranberry Jalapeño "Cornbread" Muffins

Preparation Time: 6 minutes

Cooking Time: 19 min

Serving: 8

Ingredients:

- 1 cup coconut flour
- 1/3 cup Swerve Sweetener or other erythritol
- 1 teaspoon heating powder
- 1/2 teaspoon salt
- enormous eggs, softly beaten
- 1 cup unsweetened almond milk
- 1/2 cup margarine, softened OR avocado oil
- 1/2 teaspoon vanilla
- 1 cup crisp cranberries cut down the middle
- teaspoon minced jalapeño peppers
- 1 jalapeño, seeds evacuated, cut into 12 cuts, for decorate

Directions:

1 Preheat stove to 325F and oil a biscuit tin well or line with paper liners.

2 In a medium bowl, whisk together coconut flour, sugar, heating powder, and salt. Separate any clusters with the rear of a fork.

3 Stir in eggs softened spread and almond milk and mix energetically. Mix in vanilla concentrate and keep on mixing

until blend is smooth and very much joined. Mix in slashed cranberries and jalapeños.

4   Divide player equally among arranged biscuit cups and spot one cut of jalapeño over each.

5   Bake 25 to 30 minutes or until tops are set and an analyzer embedded in the middle confesses all. Give cool 10 minutes access dish; at that point move to a wire rack to cool totally.

Nutrition:

Cal: 10, Carbs: 4g/

Net Carbs: 2.5 g,

 Fiber: 4.5 g, Fat: 8 g,

Protein: 8g, Sugars: 10 g.

50.   Keto Bagels Bread

Preparation Time: 5 minutes

Cooking Time: 17 min

Serving: 6

Ingredients:

- 1 cup (120 g) of almond flour
- 1/4 cup (28 g) of coconut flour
- 1 Tablespoon (7 g) of psyllium husk powder
- 1 teaspoon (2 g) of preparing powder
- 1 teaspoon (3 g) of garlic powder
- Pinch salt
- medium eggs (88 g)
- teaspoons (10 ml) of white wine vinegar
- 1/2 Tablespoons (38 ml) of ghee, dissolved
- 1 Tablespoon (15 ml) of olive oil
- 1 teaspoon (5 g) of sesame seeds

Directions:

1   Preheat the stove to 320°F (160°C).
2   Combine the almond flour, coconut flour, psyllium husk powder, preparing powder, garlic powder and salt in a bowl.
3   In a different bowl, whisk the eggs and vinegar together. Gradually shower in the dissolved ghee (which ought not to be steaming hot) and speed in well.

4   Add the wet blend to the dry blend and utilize a wooden spoon to join well. Leave to sit for 2-3 minutes.

5   Divide the blend into 4 equivalent measured bits. Utilizing your hands, shape the blend into a round shape and spot onto a plate fixed with material paper. Utilize a little spoon or apple corer to make the middle gap.

6   Brush the tops with olive oil and dissipate over the sesame seeds. Prepare in the broiler for 20-25 minutes until cooked through. Permit to cool marginally before getting a charge out of!

Nutrition:

Cal: 10,

Carbs: 1g/

Net Carbs: 1.5 g,

 Fiber: 2.5 g,

Fat: 8 g,

Protein: 9g,

Sugars: 3 g.

Conclusion

This book has presented you with some of the easiest and delicious bread recipes you can find. One of the most mutual struggles for anyone following the diet is that they have to cut out so many of the foods they love, like sugary foods and starchy bread products. This book helps you overcome both those issues. Focus your mindset toward the positive. Through a diet, you can help prevent diabetes, heart diseases, and respiratory problems. If you already feel pain from any of these, a diet under a doctor's supervision can greatly improve your condition. These loaves of bread are made using the normal Ingredients you can find locally, so there's no need to order anything or go to any specialty stores for any of them. With these pieces of bread, you can enjoy the same meals you used to enjoy but stay on track with your diet as much as you want. Lose the weight you want to lose, feel great, and still get to indulge in that piping hot piece of bread now and then. Spread on your favorite topping, and your bread craving will be satisfied. Moreover, we have learned that the bread machine is a vital tool to have in our kitchen. It is not that hard to put into use. All you need to learn is how it functions and what its features are. You also need to use it more often to learn the dos and don'ts of using the machine. The bread machine comes with a set of instructions that you must learn from the manual to use it the right way. There is a certain way of loading the Ingredients that must be followed, and the instructions vary according to the make and the model. So, when you first get a machine, sit down and learn the manual from start to finish; this allows you to put it to good use and get better results. !

CPSIA information can be obtained
at www.ICGtesting.com
Printed in the USA
BVHW092325270421
605944BV00004B/629